Exercise
for the Masses:
Are You Fit to Pray?

Written by
Laura Starr Levengard

Edited by Matthew Graham

Consult your physician before starting any exercise program. This is very important if you are over 35 and have been inactive for a period of time. The author and publisher disclaim any liability from loss, injury or damage, personal or otherwise, resulting from the procedures in this book.

Published by: Starpower Publishing

Visit our website: www.starpowerfitness.com

Contact: laurastarr@starpower.net

Copyright © 2011

ISBN: 978-1461199588

Printed in the United States of America

CONTENTS

INTRODUCTION

My name is Laura Starr Levengard. I have been a Certified Personal Trainer since 2002. It is my passion in this lifetime to help people in their daily lives with what is called *"functional fitness"*. This specificity helps train your body to accomplish all tasks necessary to get through the day. This may include getting in and out of bed, picking up items off of the floor, even taking care of necessary bathroom duties. This would also include participating in activities of your choosing, be it sports, driving a car or even sitting in a pew at your place of worship.

This book reviews the top five affiliated religions in the United States and is designed to educate and to be fun. My hope for this book is to be helpful and informative to invited guests of religious ceremonies and to friends, co-workers or even family members that have chosen a different path than the rest of their family or have married into a different religion.

For thousands of years, people have been praying and for just as long, people have struggled to get up off their seats or rise from kneeling. The following exercise program is designed to make you 'fit to pray' so each worshiper can concentrate fully on the mind and soul because they have already worked on their body.

WORLD RELIGION OVERVIEW

There are over 20 major religions in the world and outlined below is general overview of how a typical prayer service will go in each of the top five affiliated religions in the United States. This book is devoted to giving you easy to follow exercises to make sure that if you happen to be someone kneeling in church, you will be able to upright yourself without assistance from the pew in front of you or the person next to you. You will glean the best exercises to keep you fit and prepared to pray.

	WORLDWIDE*		**UNITED STATES****
Christianity	33%	2.1 billion	78.4%
Islam	21%	1.3 billion	0.6%
Hinduism	14%	1 billion	0.4%
Buddhism	6%	376 million	0.7%
Judaism	.22%	14 million	1.7%

* adherents.com, 2005

** The Pew Forum on Religion and Public Life: US Religious Landscape
    Survey, 2007

Christianity

A monotheistic religion which is based on the teachings of the Old Testament and Jesus of Nazareth. Many people choose to pray in church, be it Catholic or Protestant. There are over 35 types of churches in America. A typical Sunday morning service/gathering/worship will run approximately 1 – 1 ½ hours long. During a Catholic mass, you might be called upon to stand 8 times and kneel 3 times. It is not mandatory to attend church or pray daily, but prayer is suggested daily and many attend a weekly service or prayer meetings during the week.

A standard church service would generally be located in a building with wooden pews for benches. There may also be a small kneeling bench located at the foot of each row of pews.

The service calls on congregants to sit and stand multiple

times, kneel, genuflect if you are Catholic, lift prayer books and bow. Many services call for "a sign of peace" in which you would reach out and shake your neighbor's hand. For each of these actions, there are corresponding exercises to strengthen and tone the muscles used when performing the called upon tasks.

Judaism

A religion based on principles and ethics embodied in the Hebrew Bible. Many Jews pray in synagogues, where it is necessary to have a quorum of 10, called a minyan, to recite certain prayers. The service is conducted by a rabbi and may include a cantor or chazan who leads communal prayer and song.

There are six major American movements: Orthodox, Conservative, Reform, Reconstructionist, Jewish Renewal and Humanistic Judaism. The first three are the most common and are noted in order of most observant to those following a less strict observance of Jewish law.

A typical Conservative Shabbat (or Saturday) morning service will run approximately 2-3 hours long. The congregation faces the Ark, which holds the Torah, the first five books of the Jewish scriptures. Congregants and guests will stand up and sit down about 8 times. This service also calls for bowing, bending at the knees, rising on your toes and turning around. Standing fulfills an obligation for Jews to give praise to the Lord of all. Bowing acknowledges giving thanks to the King/the Holy One/God.

Buddhism

Originating in India, teaches Buddhists to lead a moral life, to be mindful and aware of thoughts and actions, and to develop wisdom and understanding. There are two major branches: Theravada ("The School of the Elders") and Mahayana ("The Great Vehicle"). In the United States, there are three major sects: Immigrant or Ethnic Buddhism, Import Buddhists, and Export or Evangelical Buddhists.

Buddhists do not pray to a Creator God, but have devotional meditation practice in temples and/or in front of shrines that can be in any location. Generally, these practices start off with an offering of rice to the monks, followed by chanting verses about morality, Buddha and the nature of the body. Meditation is in a seated position with legs crossed on a cushion that is slightly higher in the back than in the front. The entire devotional lasts just over one hour and ends with private meditation and may be followed with bowing three times from the kneeling position and touching head to ground, to the Buddha, to our Teacher and to the monks, depending on the specific sect.

Islam

A monotheistic religion originating with the teachings of Muhammad, a 7th-century Arab religious and political figure. Adherents to Islam are called Muslims and prayer for Muslims is also a spiritual experience. It reminds the individual of the presence of God in the daily activity.

Muslims pray in many locations either congregationally or individually. Many may choose to be in their homes, but the primary location is the masjid (mosque). The official religious leader of the mosque, the imam, leads services. If not present, then a leader is chosen among the worshipers according to the priority of age, degree of Quran memorizing, capacity of reciting the Quran properly. There are five prayer services each day – dawn (fajr), noon (dhuhr), mid-afternoon ('asr), sunset (maghrib) and nightfall ('isha). The amount of time is not specific, (about ten minutes each session) but related to where the sun is located in the sky.

Generally, all five prayers include many of the same body positions. Worshipers begin standing with an intention to pray, bowing and reaching hands to knees; moving to prostrate with bare forehead pressing onto floor and palms, knees, and pads of toes on floor. In between prayers, sitting upright with buttocks on the heels of both feet and hands placed on both knees. Worshipers will rise two more times and end in kneeling position.

Hinduism

A conglomeration of religious, philosophical, and cultural ideas and practices that originated in India; characterized by the belief in reincarnation. The religion calls for the belief in one Supreme Being who stands for both the creator and reality.

Worship is held in the home or in Hindu temples and led by a guru or a sage. Worship may occur up to five times a day. The three main prayers, or Aarti, occur at dawn, noon and dusk and are directed to God, to the sun and to ancestors. They last approximately 15-30 minutes long and the subsequent prayers last about 10 minutes. Instruments are often used including: kartals (finger cymbals), mridanga (a two-headed drum that can be held or carried), and harmonium (a hand-organ). Praying can be done sitting, standing, kneeling or prostrate on the floor; hands to side, clasped, up in the air or holding hands with one another. Eyes may be open or closed.

The chanting of mantras is the most popular form of worship. Yoga and meditation are also integral parts of the devotional service towards the lord. While this book does not specifically discuss yoga moves, many of the stretches are directly related to positions maintained during worship sessions.

MOVEMENTS OF A STANDARD RELIGIOUS SERVICE

Sitting, standing, kneeling, genuflecting, bowing, walking, rising up on toes, holding books, handshaking, and meditating are the standard movements.

CORRELATING MUSCLES:

Legs	Quadriceps, hamstrings, calves, buttocks - gluteus maximus/medius, inner and outer thigh - adductors and abductors
Stomach/ Back	Erector spinae, core/stomach region - rectus abdominus, obliques, and transverse abdominus, latissimus dorsi
Chest/ Shoulders/ Arms	Pectoralis, deltoids, biceps, triceps, trapezius, rotator cuff

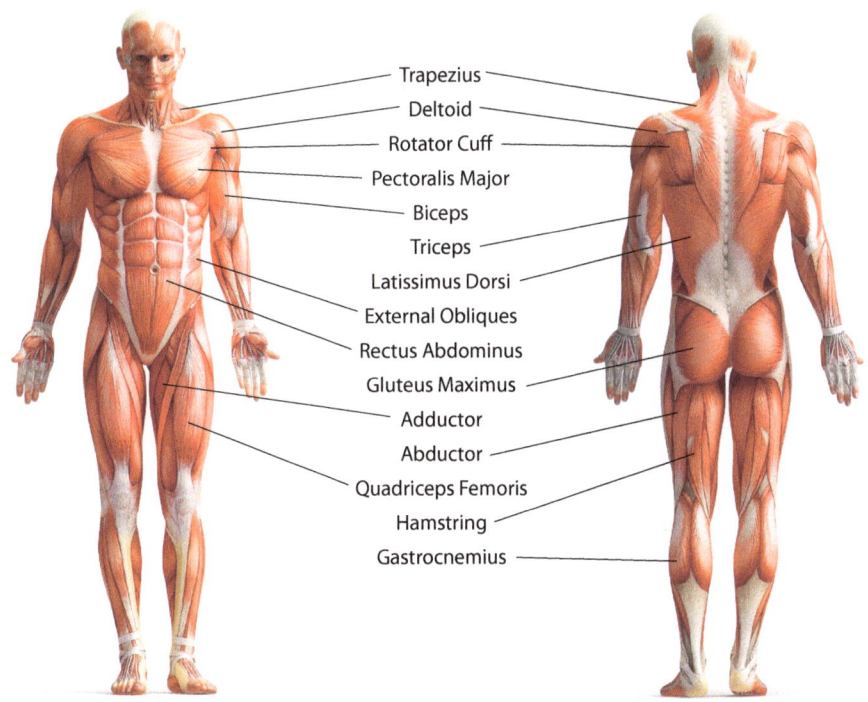

Trapezius
Deltoid
Rotator Cuff
Pectoralis Major
Biceps
Triceps
Latissimus Dorsi
External Obliques
Rectus Abdominus
Gluteus Maximus
Adductor
Abductor
Quadriceps Femoris
Hamstring
Gastrocnemius

GETTING STARTED

A complete home gym can be set up for a nominal amount. Basic equipment includes a stability ball, assorted dumbbells, stretch tubing and a yoga mat. Any clear space large enough for you to do pushups will be sufficient for you to exercise.

Stability balls are chosen according to height. If you are 5'7" or less, then choose a ball that is 55cm. 5'8" and over, use 65 cm. When you are sitting on the ball, your knees should bend at a right angle; thighs should be parallel to the floor.

Stretch or resistance tubing is a very inexpensive alternative to dumbbells. While some companies vary the color scheme, they generally are rated in strength by the color of the rainbow. They start with lighter colors to darker colors; easier to harder starting with yellow, green, red, purple, blue and black. For most of us, the greens and reds are the most useful. In this book, stretch tubing can be substituted in for most exercises where dumbbells are suggested.

Safety Tips

Warm up before exercising. You could start with a walk around the block, climbing the stairs several times or even doing a handful of jumping jacks. It is important to warm-up and 'loosen up' the muscle groups you are going to be working on that day.

Good posture or form. Stand tall, relaxed at knees and hips, keep ears over shoulders unless otherwise directed. No pain, no gain is ridiculous. If an exercise you are doing is hurting you, then stop immediately. All exercises are to be done in smooth and flowing motions. Count to 2 or 4 on each of your exercise movements to help you maintain continuity and gain the greatest benefit from each exercise.

Breathing. Of course you have to breathe! Breathe in on easy part of exercise and breathe out/exhale on more challenging part of exercise. An easy trick is to count out loud as you perform the push or pull of the exercise. You can't hold your breath when you are talking.

Once again – pain is bad. If you feel pain, then you need to stop and reevaluate what you are doing. You may need to discontinue the exercise, check your posture. A simple modification is to decrease the weight you are moving/lifting.

Recommendations from the Surgeon General on Healthy Weight Advice

If you are overweight or obese, losing just 10% of your body weight can improve your health. You can see how much, if any weight you need to lose by locating your height and weight on the body mass index (BMI) chart below.

If you need to lose weight, do so gradually-1/2 to 2 pounds per week.

Keep physically active to balance the calories you consume.

Be physically active for at least 30 minutes (adults) or 60 minutes (children) on most days of the week.

> Underweight = <18.5
> Normal weight = 18.5-24.9
> Overweight = 25-29.9
> Obesity = BMI of 30 or greater

BMI (kg/m²)	19	20	21	22	23	24	25	26	27	28	29	30	35	40
Height (inches)							Weight (lbs.)							
58	91	96	100	105	110	115	119	124	129	134	138	143	167	191
59	94	99	104	109	114	119	124	128	133	138	143	148	173	198
60	97	102	107	112	118	123	128	133	138	143	148	153	179	204
61	100	106	111	116	122	127	132	137	143	148	153	158	185	211
62	104	109	115	120	126	131	136	142	147	153	158	164	191	218
63	107	113	118	124	130	135	141	146	152	158	163	169	197	225
64	110	116	122	128	134	140	145	151	157	163	169	174	204	232
65	114	120	126	132	138	144	150	156	162	168	174	180	210	240
66	118	124	130	136	142	148	155	161	167	173	179	186	216	247
67	121	127	134	140	146	153	159	166	172	178	185	191	223	255
68	125	131	138	144	151	158	164	171	177	184	190	197	230	262
69	128	135	142	149	155	162	169	176	182	189	196	203	236	270
70	132	139	146	153	160	167	174	181	188	195	202	207	243	278
71	136	143	150	157	165	172	179	186	193	200	208	215	250	286
72	140	147	154	162	169	177	184	191	199	206	213	221	258	294
73	144	151	159	166	174	182	189	197	204	212	219	227	265	302
74	148	155	163	171	179	186	194	202	210	218	225	233	272	311
75	152	160	168	176	184	192	200	208	216	224	232	240	279	319
76	156	164	172	180	189	197	205	213	221	230	238	246	287	328

LOWER BODY EXERCISES
Sitting: Squats

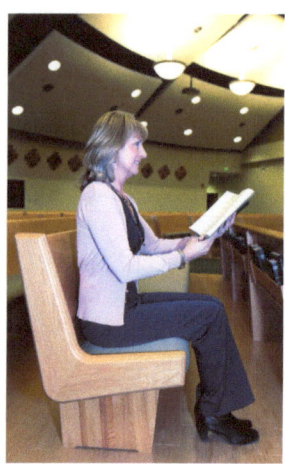 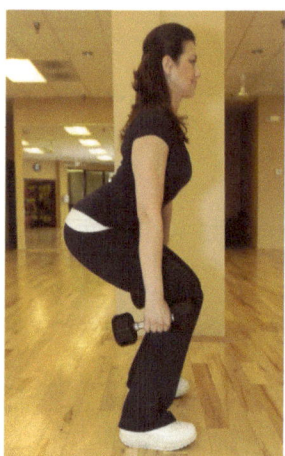

Squats performed correctly will work your quadriceps, gluteus medius and gluteus maximus (buttocks), the erector spinae (muscles surrounding the spine) and your abdominals.

1. With feet shoulder width apart and toes turned out 20-45 degrees. Keep your back as straight as possible.

2. Lower to a seated position with thighs parallel to floor and keep your knees from extending forward of your toes.

3. A chair may be used as a guide, but is not necessary.

4. Keep your heels down to prevent the knees from rocking forward beyond toes.

5. Pause in seated position and then slowly return to a standing position.

Easier: Do not lower yourself all the way.

Special Note: If you notice minor discomfort in the knees when you are squatting, turn your toes out as if in ballet class. This takes the direct pressure off of your knees and encourages strengthening more on your inner thighs to balance the larger quadriceps muscle.

Harder: Sit a little bit lower and/or hold onto some weights. You can use dumbbells or gallon-size jugs of water. These weigh approximately 8 pounds each.

Genuflection: Lunges

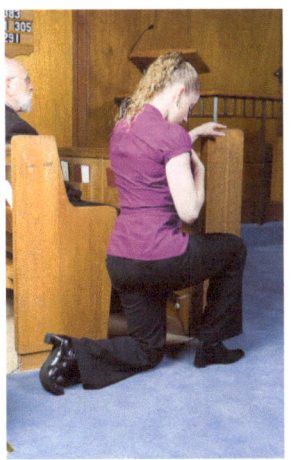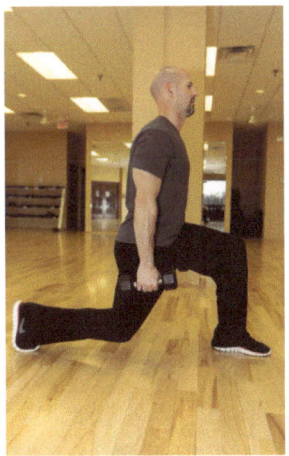

Lunges performed correctly will work your quadriceps, gluteus maximus and hamstrings. As lunges are performed, larger steps will cause the gluteus maximus to work harder and shorter steps will provide more work for the quadriceps.

1. Stand with your knees slightly flexed, one foot in front of the other, with your feet slightly farther apart than a normal step.

2. Inhale and drop the forward thigh until it is parallel to the floor and your back knee is almost touching the floor. Exhale as you return to starting position. Make sure you keep your core* engaged and lifted throughout the exercise.

3. Repeat movement with alternate leg.

* Your core consists of all of the abdominal muscles: rectus abdominus, obliques and transverse or more commonly known as your stomach. These muscles stabilize, align and move the trunk of the body. Contract your belly button in toward your spine to keep the core engaged.

Easier: Do not lower yourself so far down and/or do fewer lunges.

Harder: Hold extra weight or you can hold position for a longer period of time, say 5-10 seconds.

Bowing: Dead lifts

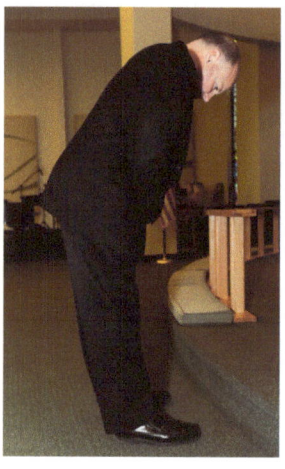 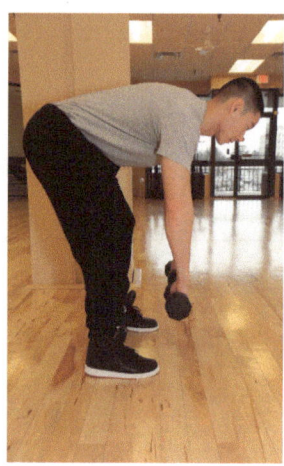

Dead lifts are a forward bending exercise to strengthen hip flexors and hamstrings.

1. Stand with feet parallel and shoulder width apart.
2. Hold weight in each hand. With head lifted and back straight, bend as far forward as possible reaching for toes. Head, neck and back should all be in a straight line.
3. Slowly return back to upright position. Less weight = less stress on lower back, so go easy in the beginning.

Easier: Do not bend as far forward and/or you could use a broom stick held in both hands while stick is parallel to floor.

Harder: Use dumbbells or gallon-size jugs of water. Full bottles of water weigh approximately 8 pounds each.

Toe Raises: Calf Raises

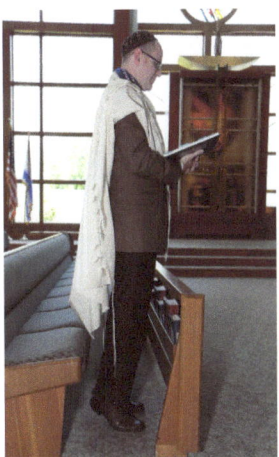 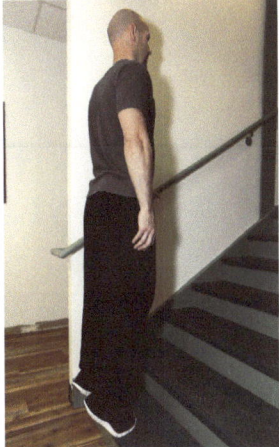 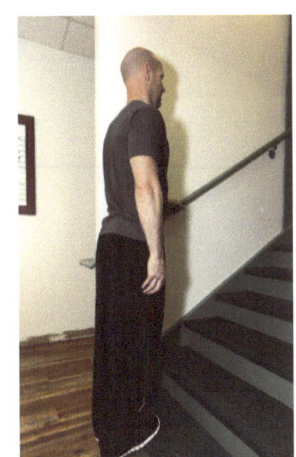

Calf raises strengthen your calves which are comprised of the gastrocnemius, soleus and anterior tibialis. Strong calves are very important in managing stairs, as well as in certain religious services, rising up on toes and getting up off the floor.

1. Standing on the first step of a flight of stairs, use the railing or wall as a guide or support if necessary.

2. Balls of feet should be on the edge of the step and heels should be off the step.

3. Rise up on to tip toes and then lower heels down below level to step. The 'work' part of this exercise is pressing up and a really good stretch is when your heels are hanging down.

Easier: Do not raise up as high.

Harder: Do raises on one foot at a time and/or hold weights at the same time.

Kneeling/Sitting/Genuflection: Side-lying Leg Raises

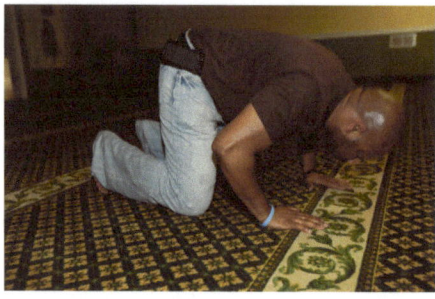 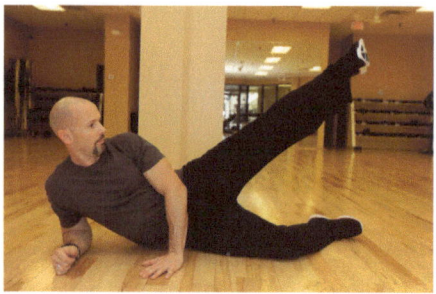

This exercise is to strengthen your inner and outer thighs (adductors and abductors).

1. For abductors, lie down on the floor on your side with legs stacked on top of each other. Upper body can be resting on forearm/elbow or all the way flat and head resting on upper arm/shoulder.

2. Slowly raise and lower the top leg with foot in flexed position (or 90 degree angle).

3. For adductors, stay in same body position, but bend top leg so that foot is flat on floor either in front or behind knee of leg on the floor.

4. Slowly raise and lower bottom leg with foot in a flexed position.

Easier: Do this exercise standing up. For abductors, stand perpendicular to a wall, feet together, place closer hand on wall and slowly extend outside leg away from the wall. For adductors, stay facing same direction, bring outside leg slightly forward and pulse towards the wall. Turn around and repeat other side.

Harder: Place a dumbbell on top leg for added resistance while doing the leg lifts or tie stretch tubing around ankles for additional challenge.

UPPER BODY EXERCISES
Sitting/Standing/Holding items: Chest Press

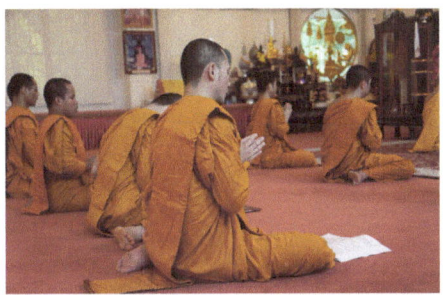

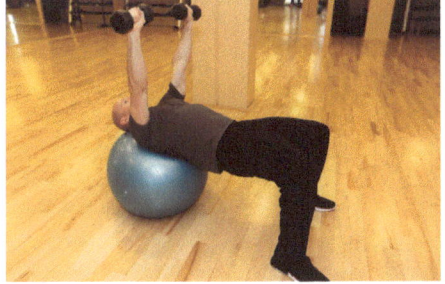
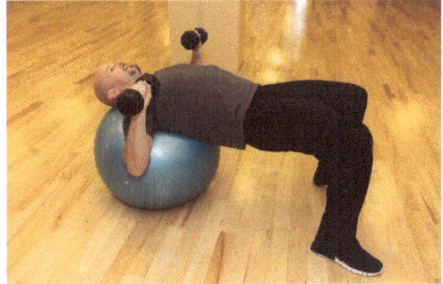

This exercise strengthens your pectorals, anterior deltoids and triceps and gives you the power to lift your arms, open and close doors and aids in your posture.

1. Using a bench, stability ball, floor or ottoman, lie down so your head, shoulders and back are supported. If you are lying on the floor, feel free to bend legs at the knees to relieve stress on low back.

2. Hold a dumbbell in each hand. Extend arms up to the ceiling, palms facing your feet with the dumbbells parallel to your chest.

3. Lower elbows almost all the way to floor or parallel to floor. Breathe in on the way down to the floor and exhale as you extend your arms up.

Easier: Lift lighter weights and/or perform exercise on one side at a time.

Harder: Use heavier weights.

Sitting/Standing/Reading: Bent Over Row

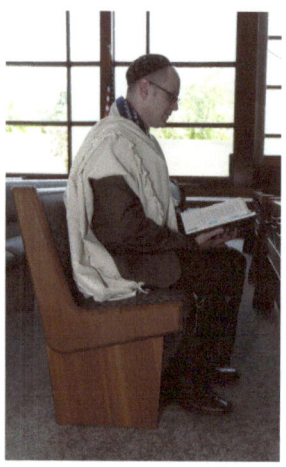 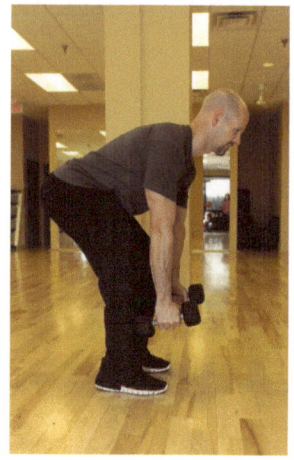 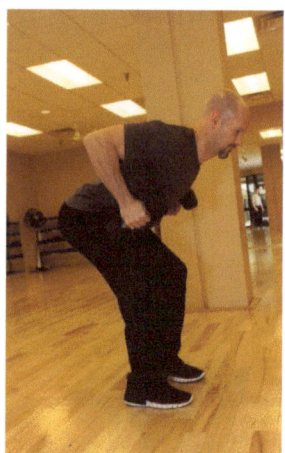

This exercise strengthens your upper back (latissimus dorsi, rhomboids and posterior deltoids) aiding you in good posture and allowing you to sit for extended time periods without stress and feeling the need to slouch forward.

1. Stand upright and hold dumbbell in each hand.
2. With knees slightly bent (commonly called 'soft knees'), bend forward from the hips keeping your back straight.
3. Arms should be hanging straight to the ground at the starting position
4. Pull the dumbbells up to your torso while keeping the elbows close to your sides.
5. Pause and then return arms to straightened position.

Easier: Use lighter weights or perform a single arm row. Place one foot forward of the other, rest same side arm on front leg and do exercise one side at a time.

Harder: Use heavier weights.

Praise/lifting of religious paraphernalia: Shoulder Presses

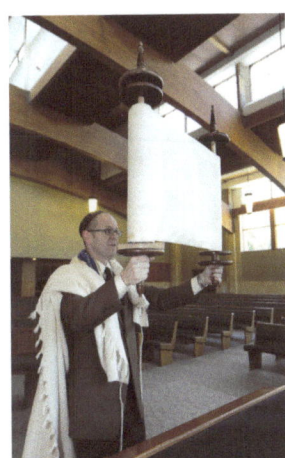 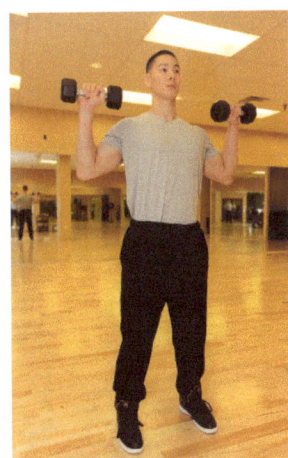 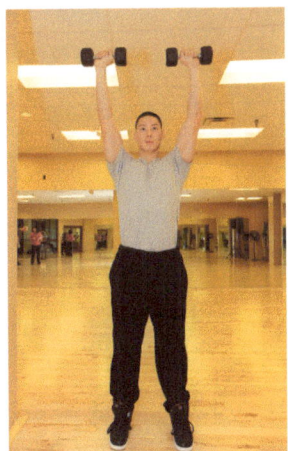

Strong shoulders mean you can lift up prayer books, crosses, babies or even just your groceries. Your shoulder muscles consist of your deltoids, trapezius and internally, the rotator cuff which is made up of 4 muscles – supraspinatus, infraspinatus, teres minor and subscapularis.

1. From a standing or sitting position on a high back chair or bench, hold weights close to your shoulders with palms facing forward. Raise your arms so that your elbows are out to the sides and at shoulder height or just slightly below. Hands should be at 12 o'clock over your elbows. Abs should be contracted for the duration of the exercise by pulling belly button to spine.

2. Breathe in as you are ready to begin. Slowly exhale as you extend your arms to the ceiling, but do not lock your elbows. At the top, your arms may come close to each other, but not touching. Not only is it not necessary to bang the weights together, it is not good 'gym etiquette.'

3. Slowly lower arms back to starting position.

Easier: Use lighter weights and/or alternate arms by extending one arm at a time.

Harder: Use heavier dumbbells.

Holding prayer book: Pushups

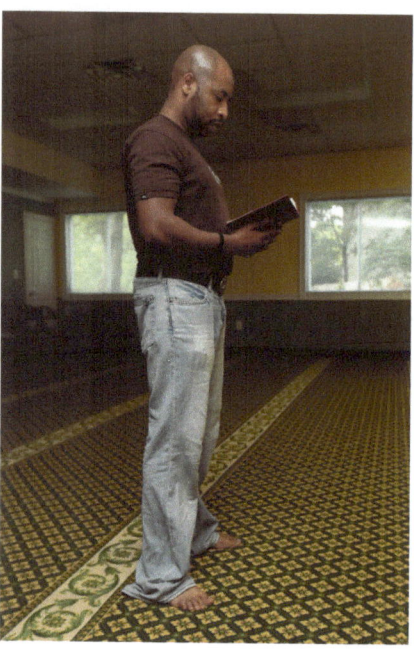
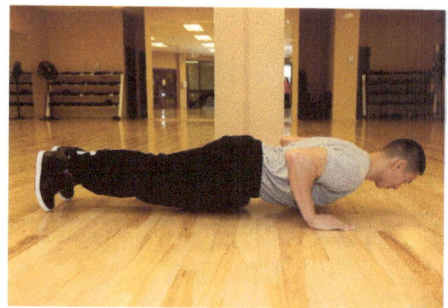
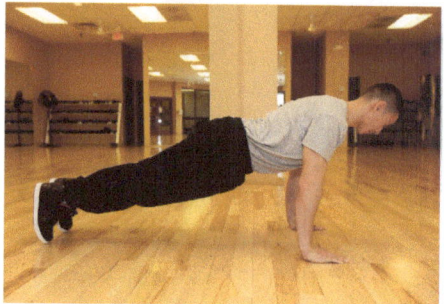

Pushups strengthen your chest – pectorals & anterior deltoids - and triceps. Similar to plank, pushups work the abdominals and back. These muscles help you carry items, not to mention help your arms look lean and strong so that when you wave, the triceps area does not continue to 'wave' when you have stopped moving your arm!

1. Place hands shoulder-width apart.

2. Keeping body straight and head not dropping down, lower chest to floor. Chest should come to about 3 inches (or one closed fist size) distance from the floor.

3. Return to starting position.

Easier: Standing with hands on wall and press in and out from wall or starting position with knees on floor.

Harder: Lift one leg off of floor or have hands closer together to form a diamond. One more option would be to have hands closer to your side and lower down for a military pushup as you direct your elbows toward your feet.

Holding a prayer book : Bicep Curls

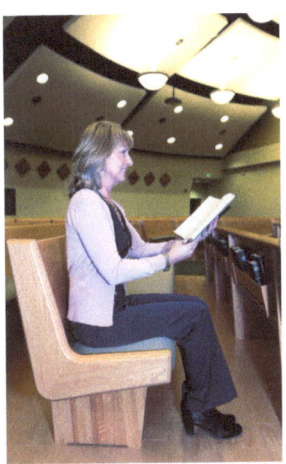 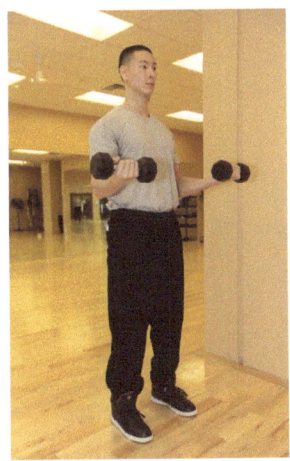 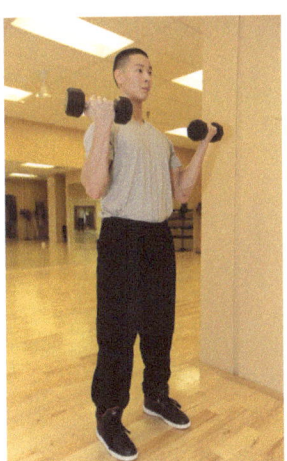

This is an isolation exercise to strengthen your biceps in your arms to better prepare you to lift and carry items, such as prayer books, Torahs, and even children.

1. Stand upright with feet shoulder width apart and knees slightly bent.

2. Form a basic curl, hold weights (dumbbells, water jugs or cans from your pantry) with palms facing out, elbows next to the body. Bend the elbows and curl the weights toward the shoulders without moving the elbows. As the lifting is the exertion/hard work part of the exercise, you should be exhaling as you lift and breathe in as you lower your arms.

3. Do not arch your back. If you can't help yourself, then decrease amount of weight or alternate arms.

4. Pause at top with weight by your shoulders and then slowly release and return to starting position with arms fully extended.

Easier: Use lighter weights or alternate arms instead of lifting both at one time.

Harder: Use heavier weights or add in a balance challenge by standing on one foot.

Handshaking/holding prayer books/raising a cross or other religious items: front and lateral (side) raises

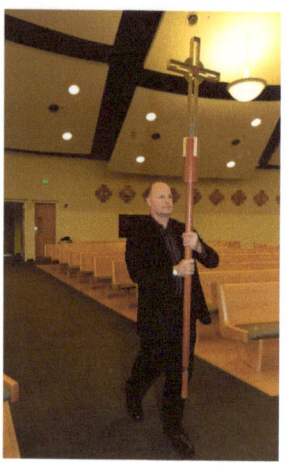 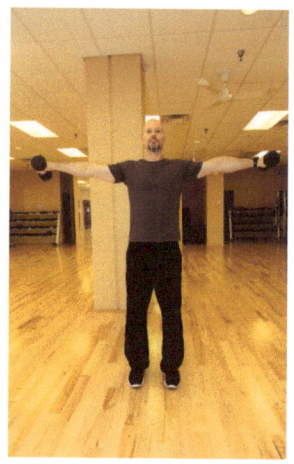 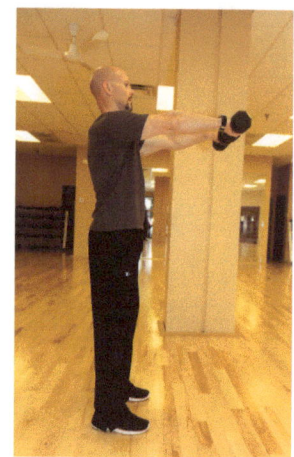

Two more excellent shoulder exercises to strengthen and help prevent injuries are front and side shoulder raises. These exercises strengthen the shoulder muscles and improve posture. This is especially important for times when you are not only sitting in a service for an extended period of time, but also for other daily activities such as working at your computer or eating meals.

1. Stand upright, knees slightly bent, arms at sides and feet shoulder width apart.

2. Holding your weights, lift straight arms directly in front of you so they end up parallel to floor at shoulder height.

3. Slowly return to starting position.

4. Side/lateral raises use the same starting position, but lift arms out to sides and end no higher than shoulder height.

Easier: Use a lighter weight or alternate arms. Try not to arch your back through the movement.

Harder: Use a heavier weight or add in a balance challenge and stand on one foot while lifting the opposite arm.

CORE EXERCISES
Standing/Sitting: Bicycle Crunches

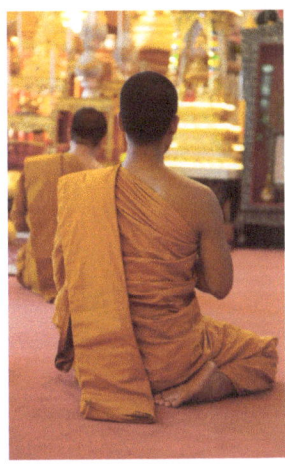 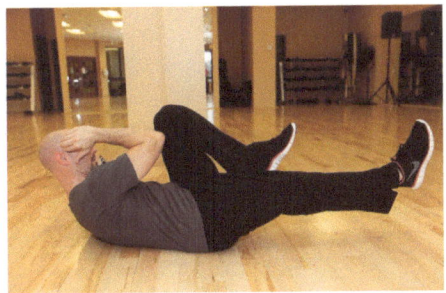

Bicycle crunches are an all encompassing core exercise that targets your rectus abdominus, obliques and transverse abdominals. This exercise is easily adaptable to be made easier or more challenging.

1. Lie down on the floor on your back.
2. Bend knees with feet on the floor and each hand alongside each ear. Touching your ears prevents you from pulling on your head and causing neck strain.
3. Use your abs/core to simultaneously bring the right knee and left shoulder toward each other. Alternate and continue in a smooth, fluid motion. The extended leg should be out as straight as possible while hovering above the floor. Shoulder blade of the reaching elbow should leave the floor.

Easier: Do not extend the leg as far out or as low over the floor.

Harder: Keep extended leg as straight as possible and come within an inch of the floor.

Sitting/Standing: Crunches and Leg Pulses

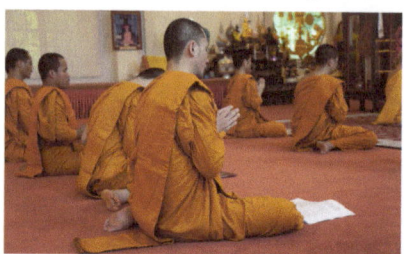

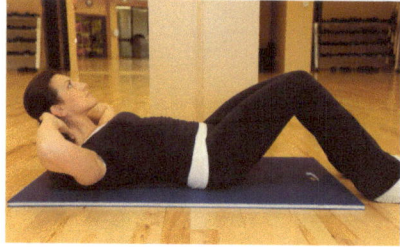 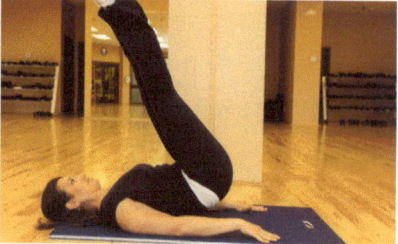

This exercise targets your rectus abdominus.

1. Lie down on floor with your knees bent and your feet flat on the floor. You can place a rolled up hand towel at the small of your back if this is an uncomfortable position for you.

2. Place hands on either side of your head and touching your ears. This position will prevent you from pulling on your head as you do exercise and keep neck pain away.

3. Breathe in deeply, then slowly exhale and lift your head, shoulders and shoulder blades up off of the floor. Slowly return to floor.

4. After set of crunches is finished, remove towel if used and extend legs straight up to the ceiling. Place hands palms down on the floor or under your tailbone.

5. Slowly press your feet to the ceiling as you lift your lower body a couple of inches off of the floor. This works best when you pull your belly button toward your spine and contract your abs. Return and repeat.

6. When finished, hug your knees into your chest. Ahh!

Easier: Do not lift as far off the ground.

Harder: Lift up higher off the ground when doing either the upper crunch or lower crunch. Even more challenging would be to lift upper and lower at the same time.

Standing/Sitting: Plank

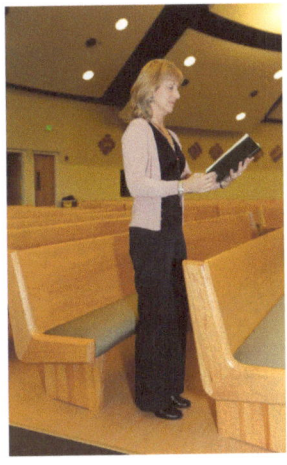 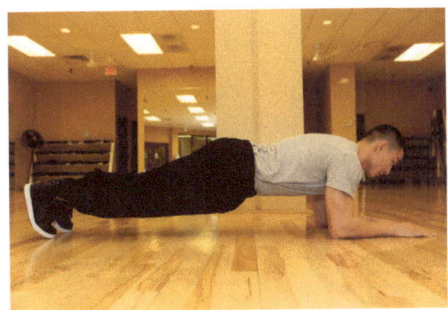

The plank is an all-over exercise that works your arms, back, abdomen, legs. Core strength is critical to help maintain proper posture and reduce back pain. Religious services can tend to be rather lengthy; having this physical strength can let you focus on your prayers. The saying goes "a strong stomach, a strong back."

1. Lie face down on mat with elbows resting on floor next to chest.
2. Push your body off the floor in a pushup position with body resting on elbows or hands. Contract the abs and keep the body in a straight line from head to toes. Hold for 30-60 seconds and repeat as many times as you can.

Easier: Start on your knees and progress to one knee off the floor, then both.

Harder: Lift one foot up off the floor for half the duration, then switch.

Sitting/Standing/Bowing: Side Plank

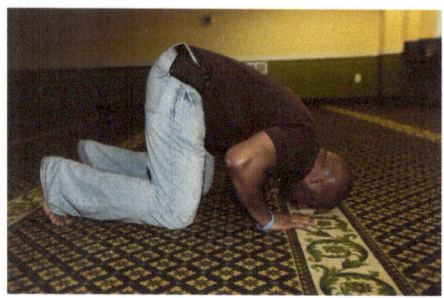 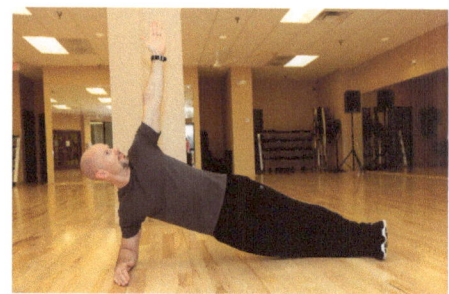

The side plank is an all-over exercise that works primarily your obliques, arms, back, abdomen, legs. Core strength is critical to help maintain proper posture and reduce back pain.

1. Begin by lying on your side, propped up on elbow. Feet, hips and knees should be stacked on top of each other.

2. Lift hips off of floor, while balancing on stacked feet and pressing forearm into floor. Use top hand on floor to gain initial balance is acceptable, but as soon as you are steady, place that hand along your side or reach for ceiling.

3. Concentrate on pulling belly button into spine all while maintaining your balance. Strive for 30-60 seconds in this position.

Easier: Bend lower leg and use bottom knee for support.

Harder: Raise top leg while in side plank position or you can add movement by taking top arm and swinging it down in front of you and ultimately reaching through and back up.

Sitting/Standing: Knee Up

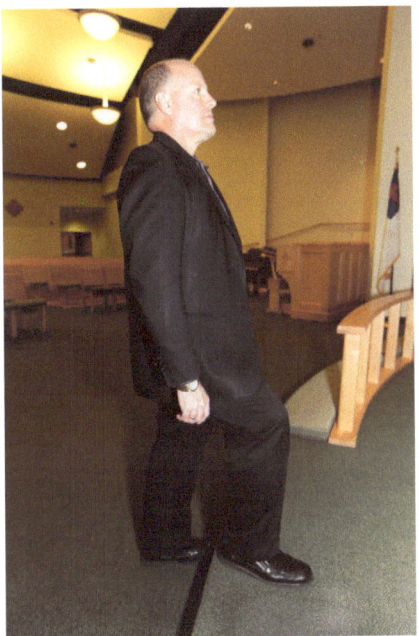
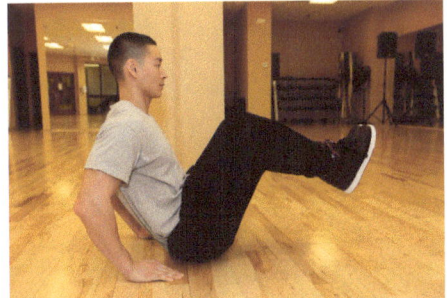
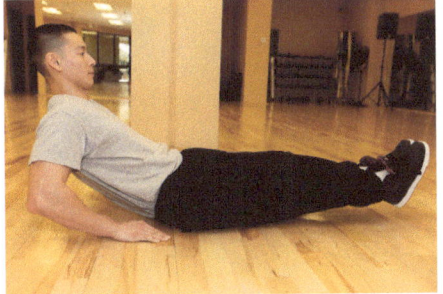

This exercise focuses on core stability and balance.

1. Begin seated on floor with knees up and feet flat on floor.
2. Place hands on floor with fingers pointing straight ahead toward toes and lean slightly back to the point of feeling your abdominals working to hold you upright.
3. Lift feet off floor with knees directed toward chest.
4. Slowly extend legs parallel to floor with heels a few inches off the floor. You should breathe in as you extend and exhale as you compress back to beginning.
5. Slowly bring knees back to your chest.
6. Repeat exercise for 10-15 repetitions.

Easier: Do not lower legs to completely parallel and keep legs slightly bent.

Harder: Lift hands off the floor and reach for the ceiling as you raise and lower legs.

Sitting/Standing: Windshield Wipers

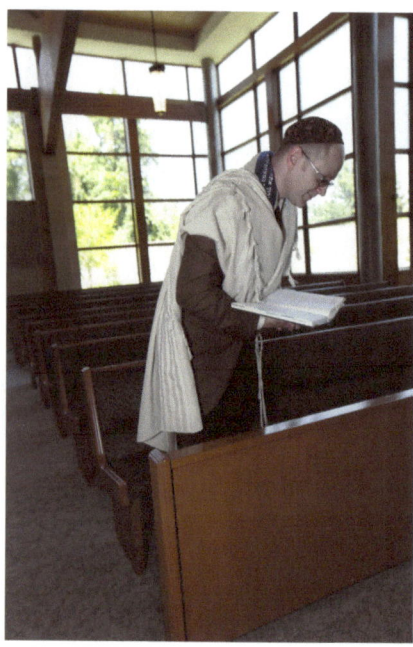
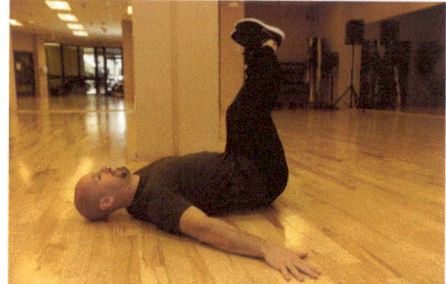
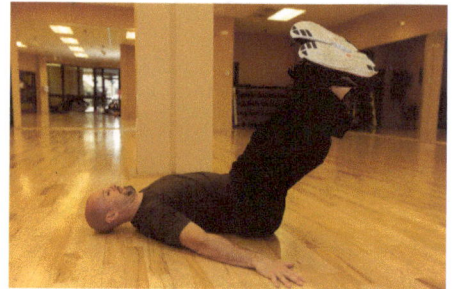

This exercise primarily targets the obliques.

1. Lie down flat on back with legs extended up to the ceiling.
2. With hands on floor at your side, slowly lower legs to the left, raise and lower to the right. You can think of this as if your legs are the windshield wipers on your car that sweep from side to side.

Easier: Do not lower legs as far. If your legs are like the arms on a clock – move left and right from 11 to 1 or 10 to 2. You can also have legs bent at knee in a 90 degree angle.

Harder: Drop legs low to the ground while trying to maintain keeping hips/butt planted on floor. Think of your legs moving from noon down to 9 and then rotate over to 3.

Sitting/Standing/Bowing: Writing the ABC's

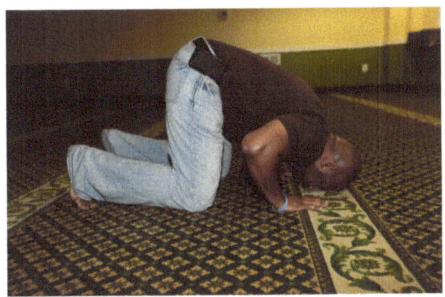 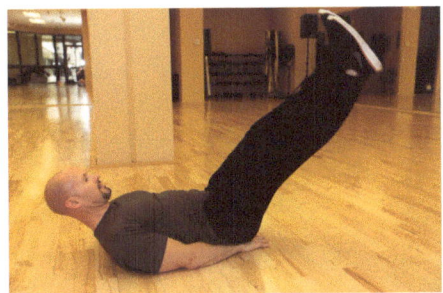

This exercise primarily targets the obliques and rectus abdominus.

1. Lie down flat on back with legs extended up to the ceiling.

2. With hands on floor at your side or under your hips, slowly lower the legs together as one unit to write out the alphabet from A-Z. Consider 'writing' letters in cursive capital letters for smooth flow.

Easier: Do not lower legs as far. Making smaller letters is easier.

Harder: Write your letters very big all while trying to maintain the hips/butt planted on floor.

STRETCHES

Stretching is very important for injury prevention, flexibility, increased range of motion, quicker recovery from exercise and stress relief. Stretching during exercise can be done initially before you begin workout, after each exercise is performed or at the end of your fitness session. Stretching can be done up to three times per muscle and held for 30-60 seconds each.

When you stretch, you stretch the opposite of direction of the exercise performed. For example, if you do a bicep curl, the corresponding stretch would be to extend your arm straight out and gently pulling the arm back toward the body. More examples and pictures are just ahead!

Neck Stretch

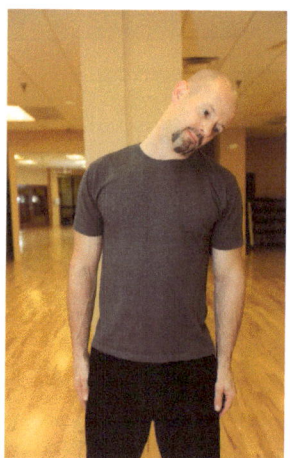

1. Standing comfortably with feet shoulder width apart, hands along side, tilt head to right reaching ear to shoulder.
2. Hold for 30 seconds.
3. Roll head toward chest and end up with left ear just over the left shoulder.

** Never roll head around the back, only to the front! There is a significant potential for neck injury if performed incorrectly. **

Back Stretch/Posterior Deltoid Stretch

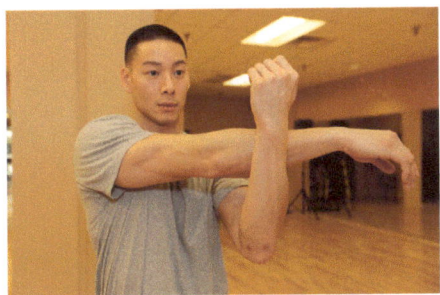

1. Extend right arm straight out in front of you at chest height.

2. Take left arm and gently pull right arm across the front of your body. Make sure to keep standing or sitting straight up.

3. Release after 30 seconds and repeat on opposite side.

Chest Stretch/Pectoralis Major Stretch

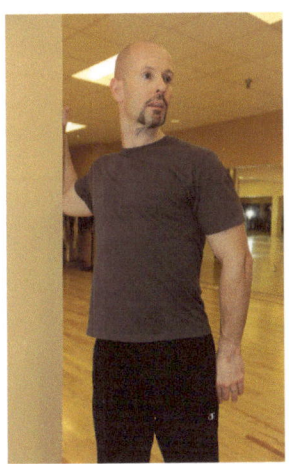

1. From standing position, place hand or forearm on a wall or doorframe at chest height or slightly below.

2. Extend arm as far as you can and begin to twist your body away from wall. Look in the direction that you are turning.

3. Hold for 30 seconds and repeat opposite side.

Bicep Stretch

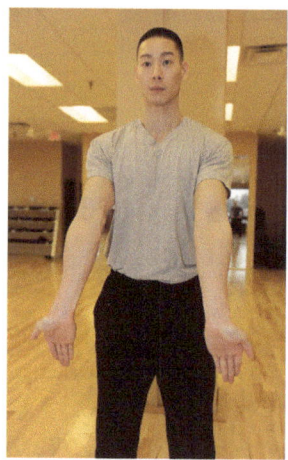

1. Hold both arms outstretched in front of you with palms face up to ceiling.

2. Extend fingers as far as you can and while arms are still reaching out, reach fingers down toward the floor.

Triceps Stretch

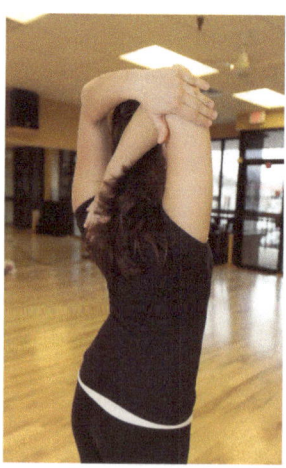

1. From standing or sitting position, extend one arm up over head. Bend arm at elbow and drop hand behind your head.

2. With opposite hand, grab elbow and gently pull arm downwards.

3. Hold stretch for 30 seconds and repeat opposite side.

Side Stretch

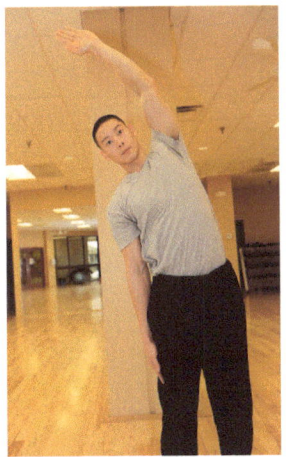

1. Begin in standing position, feet comfortably apart.

2. Reach both hands straight up to ceiling and then drop one arm down along side.

3. Continue to reach one arm up to ceiling and lean slightly so the arm reaches over toward opposite side. Hold for 30 seconds.

4. Repeat on opposite side

Quadriceps Stretch

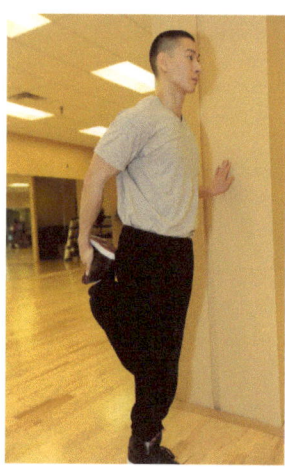

1. Stand comfortably on both legs. Have a chair or wall nearby for support just in case. This stretch is also excellent for working on your balancing skills.

2. Balancing on one leg, bend opposite leg at the knee with the foot reaching for your buttocks. Grab chair if necessary with one hand and grab your foot with the other.

3. Gently pull heel to buttocks while pressing hips forward. Keep knees as close together as possible.

4. Hold for 30 seconds and then gently release.

5. Repeat on opposite side.

Hamstring Stretch

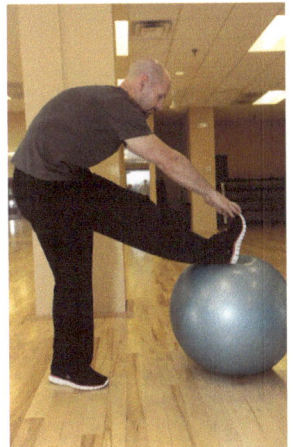
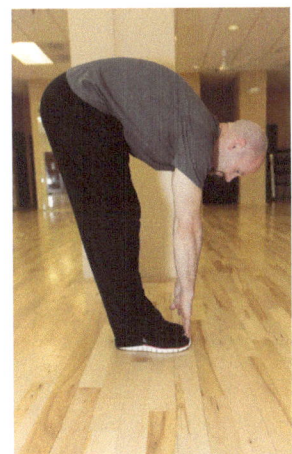

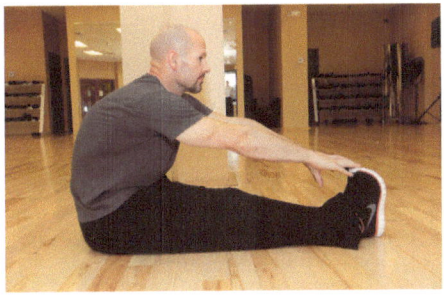

This stretch can be performed multiple ways and you can decide which the best stretch is.

Version 1 – standing with feet together, bend forward at the hips and reach for toes, keeping your legs straight. Do not let the knees bend.

Version 2 – place one foot up on a chair or bench. Bend at hip and reach forward to toes.

Version 3 – sitting on floor with legs extended in front of you, bend at hips and reach forward for toes.

Hold stretch for 30 seconds.

Calf Stretch

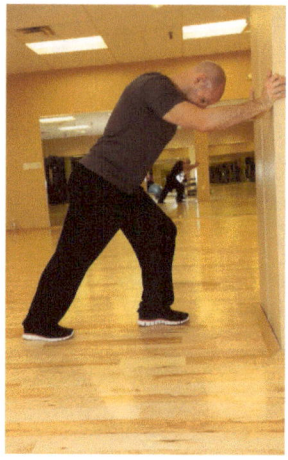

1. Standing with feet slightly apart and one foot forward of the other, place hands on a wall or the back of a chair.

2. Bend forward knee slightly, straighten back leg and press heel into floor.

3. Hold for 30 seconds and repeat opposite side.

Lower Back and Stomach – Cat and Cow Stretch/ Child's pose

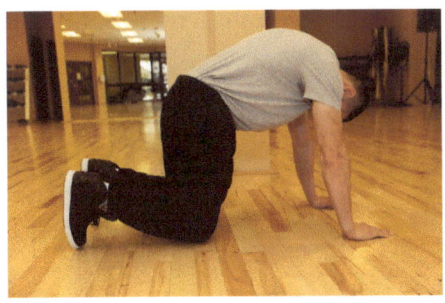
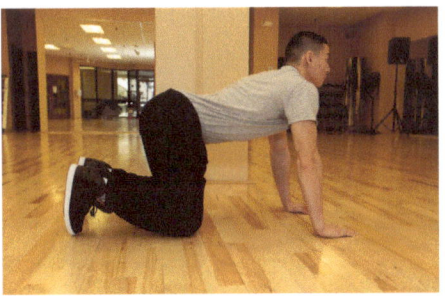
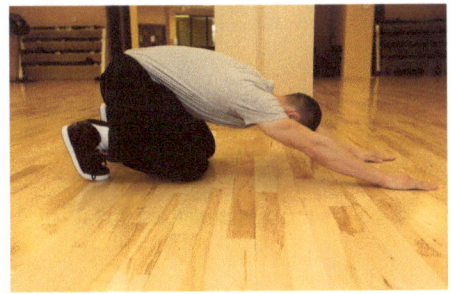

1. Begin on hands and knees.
2. Inhale and arch back up to ceiling while lowering head to floor.
3. Exhale, look up and drop belly towards floor.
4. Repeat 2-3 times.
5. Finish by sitting your butt back towards your heels.

WORKOUT ROUTINES

Warm up for a few minutes with a light jog or by marching in place. You may also jump rope or perform jumping jacks. This is to warm up your muscles and get them ready for strength training. This is especially helpful if you plan to exercise first thing in the morning.

Goal: 3 sets of 12-15 repetitions (reps)

Do each of this one time through as one set.

Take a one minute rest period in between sets; choose one of the following depending on if you are working lower or upper body exercises:

> Walk around and have a water break
> Jog in place
> Jumping Jacks
> Quadriceps stretch – 30 seconds each leg for a total of one minute for break
> Hamstring stretch for one minute
> Bicep Stretch
> Chest Stretch
> Back Stretch

Routine #1

Lunges – can do all of one side at a time or alternate legs
Squats
Bicycle Crunches

Push ups
Bent Over Row
Bicep Curls
Windshield Wipers

Chest Press
Shoulder Press
Lateral Raises
Knee Up

Goal: 3 sets of 12-15 repetitions (reps)

Workout Notes

_____

_____

_____

_____

_____

_____

_____

_____

Workout Routine #2

Squats
Deadlifts
Calf Raises
Bicycle Crunches

Chest Press
Lateral Raises
Front Raises
Plank

Bent Over Row
Push Ups
Bicep Curls
Windshield Wipers

Goal: 3 sets of 12-15 repetitions (reps)

Workout Notes

_____

_____

_____

_____

_____

_____

_____

_____

Workout Routine #3

Squats
Lunges – stationary or walk across the room and come back
Side-lying leg raises
Crunches alternating with leg pulses

Chest Press
Bent Over Row
Bicep Curl
Side Plank

Push Ups
Shoulder Press
Front Raise
Write ABC's

Goal: 3 sets of 12-15 repetitions (reps)

Workout Notes

_____

_____

_____

_____

_____

_____

_____

_____

CONCLUDING THOUGHTS AND SUGGESTIONS

Grab a pedometer and start walking! The Surgeon General recommends 10,000 steps per day and that equals approximately 5 miles. Park a little farther from your destination, take the stairs instead of the elevator, whatever you need to do to just get up and get moving!

Make sure to stay hydrated every day. Drink 64 oz. (or 8 cups) per day. Keep a water bottle with you at all times and try to choose water as your drink of choice with meals.

Remember – stretch every day, do weight or strength-training 2-4 times per week and cardio (walking, bike riding, elliptical, swimming) at least 3 times per week. Try a water/pool class, try a yoga class, sign up for dance. You could even hula hoop! There are so many choices for exercise. Find something you like and keep at it!

Wishing you peace, comfort, strength and ease in your future. Thank you for reading.

Laura

About the Author

Laura Starr Levengard has been a personal trainer since February 2002. She has personal trainer certifications with American Council on Exercise and Aerobics and Fitness Association of America. With several hundred continuing education credit hours under her belt, Laura has also attained Certified Instructor status for Healthy Moms® Pre/Postnatal Fitness Programs, Resist-a-Ball®, Gliding ™, Body Bar ™ and Smart Bells®. One of her specialties is balance training and she is a Master Trainer for BOSU® since 2006, teaching the teachers in the Mid-Atlantic region.

Looking for a speaker?

Laura has trained thousands of men, women and children and has been an invited speaker to numerous organizations over the years. Laura would be happy to speak to any congregation or gathering on health and wellness. Laura's frank and honest approach to fitness is results-oriented and makes exercise accessible and fun for everybody.

To have Laura speak to your congregation or community group or conduct a fitness workshop, please email laurastarr@starpower.net.

CREDITS

I wish to thank the following:

Religious advisors:
Reverend Patricia S. Downing, Rabbi Janet Ozur Bass, Mimi I. Hassanein, Swami Atmajnanananda, Shanthi Chandra Sekar, Abdul-latif Sawah and Rabbi Howard Gorin.

Editor for many a reading and review:
Matthew Graham

Accountability partner:
Marcie Lovett for our weekly phone calls and helping me learn so much in the publication/marketing arena.

Host religious venues:
The Lutheran Church of Saint Andrew, Wat Thai DC Buddhist Temple, The Islamic Society of the Washington Area all in Silver Spring, MD and Har Shalom in Potomac, MD

Fitness models:
Graham Harding, Anna Lysetskaya, Steve Truong

Religious models:
Greg Twombley, Wendy Linstrom, Hazzan Henrique Ozur Bass, Abdul Kabba and the resident Monks from Wat Thai DC Buddhist Temple

Special thanks to my family and friends for their encouragement.

Photo credits:
Ellen Cohan Photography – cover photo of Laura Levengard
Marc Warshawsky – all model photos

Layout and design:
Robyn Shrater Seemann/RS2 Studio